Making health services adolescent friendly

Developing national quality standards for adolescent friendly health services

Department of Maternal, Newborn, Child and Adolescent Health

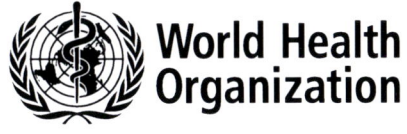

Acknowledgements

One of the key recommendations made at the Global Consultation on Adolescent Friendly Health Services organized by WHO in 2001 was to develop tools to support countries in improving the quality of health service provision to adolescents.

In line with this, WHO set out to develop a tool that countries could use to define quality standards for health services.

Save the Children, UK seconded Siobhan Peattie to WHO for six months in 2002, to contribute to the development of these tools. She worked with staff from the former Department of Child and Adolescent Health and Development to organize a meeting, drawing on the ideas and suggestions of various stakeholders and, based on this, developed the first draft of the tool.

Following further discussions, it was agreed that before finalizing the tool, it would need to undergo reality testing. It was decided to use it in draft form to support countries and to use these experiences to strengthen it. Between 2002 and 2012, the tool was used to develop national quality standards for adolescent-friendly health services in dozens of countries in all five WHO regions. WHO staff from headquarters (Paul Bloem, Krishna Bose and Jane Ferguson) and staff from the WHO Regional Offices (Matilde Maddaleno, AMRO; Nagbandja Kampatibe, AFRO; Valentina Baltag, EURO; Neena Raina, SEARO; and Patanjali Nayar, WPRO) used the tool and contributed to its further development. Staff from ministries of health and nongovernmental organizations in countries around the world also did so.

The main lesson emerging from these experiences was that while the overall objective of developing national quality standards for adolescent-friendly health services would remain unchanged, the way in which this is done varies depending on the context. In light of this, the tool underwent many changes over time that contributed to making it leaner and more flexible.

Dr Venkatraman Chandra-Mouli oversaw the development of the tool from the concept stage to the finished product.

WHO Library Cataloguing-in-Publication Data

Making health services adolescent friendly: developing national quality standards for adolescent friendly health services.

1.Adolescent health services – standards. 2.Adolescent health services – organization and administration. 3.National health programs. 4.Adolescent. I.World Health Organization.

ISBN 978 92 4 150359 4   (NLM classification: WA 330)

© **World Health Organization 2012**

All rights reserved. Publications of the World Health Organization are available on the WHO web site (www.who.int) or can be purchased from WHO Press, World Health Organization, 20 Avenue Appia, 1211 Geneva 27, Switzerland (tel.: +41 22 791 3264; fax: +41 22 791 4857; e-mail: bookorders@who.int). Requests for permission to reproduce or translate WHO publications – whether for sale or for noncommercial distribution – should be addressed to WHO Press through the WHO web site (http://www.who.int/about/licensing/copyright_form/en/index.html).

The designations employed and the presentation of the material in this publication do not imply the expression of any opinion whatsoever on the part of the World Health Organization concerning the legal status of any country, territory, city or area or of its authorities, or concerning the delimitation of its frontiers or boundaries. Dotted lines on maps represent approximate border lines for which there may not yet be full agreement. The mention of specific companies or of certain manufacturers' products does not imply that they are endorsed or recommended by the World Health Organization in preference to others of a similar nature that are not mentioned. Errors and omissions excepted, the names of proprietary products are distinguished by initial capital letters.

All reasonable precautions have been taken by the World Health Organization to verify the information contained in this publication. However, the published material is being distributed without warranty of any kind, either expressed or implied. The responsibility for the interpretation and use of the material lies with the reader. In no event shall the World Health Organization be liable for damages arising from its use.

Design by Inís Communication – www.iniscommunication.com
Printed in Switzerland

Contents

Abbreviations Iv

Introduction V

Chapter 1 1

Chapter 2 10

Chapter 3 18

Annex 1 30

Annex 2 38

Abbreviations

Abbreviations

AFHS	adolescent-friendly health services
AIDS	acquired immune deficiency syndrome
HIV	human immunodeficiency virus
HSDP	health service delivery point
NGO	nongovernmental organization
RH	reproductive health
STI	sexually transmitted infection
UNFPA	United Nations Population Fund
UNICEF	United Nations Children's Fund
WHO	World Health Organization

Introduction

This Guidebook sets out the public health rationale for making it easier for adolescents to obtain the health services that they need to protect and improve their health and well-being, including sexual and reproductive health services. It defines 'adolescent-friendly health services' from the perspective of quality, and provides step-by-step guidance on developing quality standards for health service provision to adolescents. Drawing upon international experience, it is also tailored to national epidemiological, social, cultural and economic realities, and provides guidance on identifying what actions need to be taken to assess whether appropriate standards have been achieved.

The Guidebook is intended to be a companion to the *Quality Assessment Guidebook: A guide to assessing health services for adolescent clients*, which was published by the World Health Organization (WHO) in 2009. These two guidebooks are part of a set of tools to standardize and scale up the coverage of quality health services to adolescents, as described in another WHO publication: *Strengthening the health sector's response to adolescent health and development*.

The current publication is intended for national public health programme managers, and individuals in organizations supporting their work. Its focus is on managers working in the government sector, but it will be equally relevant to those working in nongovernmental organizations (NGOs) and in the commercial sector.

Chapter 1 outlines the theoretical basis for actions to improve the quality of health service provision to adolescents. It covers the following issues and themes:

The meaning of the terms 'adolescents', 'health' and 'health services'.

- What adolescents need to grow and develop in good health.
- The role of health service provision in contributing to the health and development of adolescents.
- Main health problems of adolescents.
- Whom adolescents typically turn to for help when they face health problems;
- the factors that make it difficult for adolescents to obtain the health services they need.

- What adolescents perceive as 'friendly' health services.
- What is currently being done to make health services adolescent-friendly.
- Evidence of the effectiveness of actions to improve the provision and use of health services (in relation to adolescents).
- WHO recommendations for reaching adolescents with essential health services.

Chapter 2 describes a step-by-step process to develop national quality standards for health service provision to adolescents. It explains the importance of each of the following five steps and describes how they can be undertaken:

- Developing a shared understanding of adolescent health and of strengthening health service provision to adolescents.
- Establishing the basis for formulating the national quality standards for health service provision to adolescents, in national HIV and/or reproductive health policies and strategies.
- Developing the national standards.
- Examining the programmatic implications of applying national quality standards.
- Outlining the preparatory work that needs to be done at a national level before quality standards can be applied.

Chapter 3 provides materials that can be used to prepare for and conduct a workshop to develop national quality standards for adolescent-friendly health services. It contains:

- The outline of a background paper for a national workshop to develop national quality standards on adolescent-friendly health services.
- The objectives and agenda for a workshop to develop national quality standards for adolescent-friendly health services, and a facilitators guide to conduct the workshop.
- A set of slides for the facilitator to use in conducting the workshop.

Annex 1 lists the five dimensions of quality health services for adolescents and the twenty characteristics that relate to them.

Annex 2 lists the actions to be taken at national, district and local levels to improve the quality of health service provision to adolescents.

CHAPTER 1

A quality framework for improving the provision and use of health services, including sexual and reproductive health services, by adolescents

Outline

1. What do we mean by the term 'adolescents'?
2. What do we mean by the term 'health'?
3. What do adolescents need in order to grow and develop in good health?
4. What do we mean by the term 'health services'?
5. What is the role of health service provision in contributing to the health and development of adolescents?
6. What are the main health problems of adolescents?
7. When adolescents face health problems whom do they turn to for help?
8. What are the factors that make it difficult for adolescents to obtain the health services they need?
9. What do adolescents perceive as 'friendly' health services?
10. What is currently being done to make health services adolescent-friendly?
11. What is the evidence of the effectiveness of actions to improve the provision and utilization of health services (in relation to adolescents)?
12. What can be done to improve the quality of health service provision to adolescents?
13. What can be done to ensure that high quality health services reach all the adolescents who need them?

What do we mean by the term 'adolescents'?

Adolescence, or the second decade of life, is a period in which an individual undergoes major physical and psychological changes. Alongside this, there are enormous changes in social interactions and relationships. It is a phase in an individual's life rather than a fixed time period; a phase in which an individual is no longer a child but is not yet an adult.[1]

---

1 *The health of young people: A challenge and a promise.* Geneva, World Health Organization, 1993.

Adolescence is a time of opportunity, but also one of risk. It presents a window of opportunity because actions could be taken during this period to set the stage for healthy adulthood and to reduce the likelihood of problems in the years that lie ahead (e.g. prevention of cardiovascular diseases of adulthood through the development of healthy eating and exercising habits). At the same time, it is a period of risk; a period when health problems that have serious immediate consequences can and do occur (such as deaths resulting from road traffic injuries, and sexually transmitted infections and unwanted pregnancies resulting from unprotected sexual activity); a period when problem behaviours which could have serious adverse effects on health in the future (such as tobacco smoking and alcohol consumption) are initiated.

Adolescents are a diverse group. For example, a boy of twelve is at a very different stage of personal development than a boy of eighteen. Similarly, in addition to the obvious physical differences, he is different in psychological and social terms from a girl of the same age. A boy of twelve who is fending for himself on the street is likely to be growing and developing very differently from a boy of a similar age who is growing up with a caring and financially secure family. Even two boys of the same age, growing up in very similar circumstances, may grow and develop in different ways and time lines.

What do we mean by the term 'health'?

WHO's constitution defines health as: "a state of complete physical, mental and social well-being and not merely the absence of disease or infirmity."[2] This definition, which includes the absence of disease or infirmity on the one hand and well-being on the other, is as relevant today as it was when it was formulated in 1948.

What do adolescents need in order to grow and develop in good health?

In 1995, WHO, in conjunction with the United Nations Children's Fund (UNICEF) and the United Nations Population Fund (UNFPA), agreed on a *Common Agenda for Action* in adolescent health and development. This common agenda has the twin goals of promoting healthy development in adolescents, and the prevention of and response to health problems if and when they arise. It calls for the implementation of a package of interventions, tailored to meet the special needs and problems of adolescents, which includes the provision of information and skills, the creation of a safe and supportive environment, and the provision of health and counselling services.[3]

A useful analogy is that of an 8 year-old girl who needs to cross the road every day to get to school. She needs information and skills: on where to look, what to look for, when to walk across, and when not to do so. She needs a safe and supportive environment: a pedestrian crossing, traffic lights that work or a traffic warden in position, drivers who respect traffic rules or are punished if they do not do so. She may also need health and counselling services, if she stumbles and falls, or is struck down by a vehicle.

---

2 *Constitution of the World Health Organization.* Geneva, World Health Organization, 1948.

3 *WHO, UNFPA, UNICEF. Common agenda for action in adolescent health and development.* Geneva, World Health Organization, 1997.

Who needs to contribute to helping them grow and develop in good health? What is the special contribution that health workers and health services within this?

Many individuals and institutions have important contributions to make to the health and development of adolescents. It may be useful to think of them in concentric circles of contact and influence. At the centre is the adolescent himself or herself. Parents, siblings and close family members are in daily contact with the adolescent and constitute the first circle. The second circle includes people in regular contact with them such as their own friends, family friends, teachers, religious leaders and others. The third circle includes musicians, film stars and sports figures who have a tremendous influence on them, from afar. Finally in the fourth circle, politicians, journalists and bureaucrats, business magnates and others affect their lives in small and big ways, through their words and deeds.

What do we mean by the term health services? And what is the role of health services in contributing to the health and development of adolescents?

By health services, we mean a service provided by a health worker to a patient aimed at preventing a health problem, or detecting and treating one. It often includes the provision of information, advice and counselling.

As indicated above, health workers are part of the list of players who need to contribute to the health and development of adolescents. They have two complementary roles to play. Firstly, as service providers, they have important contributions to make in helping well adolescents stay well, and in helping ill adolescents get back to good health.

They do this through:

- the provision of information, advice, counselling and clinical services aimed at promoting health and preventing health problems and problem behaviours;
- the diagnosis, detection and management of health problems and problem behaviours; and
- referral to other health and social service providers, when necessary.
- Health workers have another important role to play – that of change agents in their communities. They have credibility and influence in their communities and need to use this to help influential community members take adolescent health seriously. They could make an invaluable contribution in helping educators, religious leaders, political leaders and others understand the needs of adolescents, and the importance of working together to meet these needs.[4]

---

4 *Programming for adolescent health and development. Report of a WHO/UNFPA/UNICEF study group on programming for adolescent health.* Geneva, World Health Organization, 1999.

What are the health problems that adolescents experience?

Many adolescents make the transition to adulthood in good health. Many others do not and may face some of the health problems[5,6] listed below:

- injuries resulting from accidents or violence;
- mental health problems;
- problems resulting from substance use;
- sexual and reproductive health problems (e.g. too-early pregnancy, mortality and morbidity during pregnancy and child birth including due to unsafe abortion, sexually transmitted infections including HIV, harmful traditional practices such as female genital mutilation, and sexual coercion);
- problems resulting from under nutrition and over nutrition;
- endemic diseases (e.g. tuberculosis and malaria).

Some of these health problems affect the individual during adolescence (e.g. a death caused by suicide or interpersonal violence or from the consequences of an unsafe abortion). Others affect the individual later in life (e.g. lung cancer resulting from tobacco use initiated during adolescence).

When adolescents have health-related concerns or are experiencing health problems to whom do they turn for help?[7]

As indicated above, most adolescents make the transition into adulthood in good health (although some of them do not). Those adolescents who are well tend to see no good reason for visiting a health facility. (In most developing countries, the system of periodic check-ups to monitor progress is limited to children under the age of five, and to pregnant women). Those adolescents who fall ill with, for example, commonly occurring conditions such as fevers, coughs and colds, may have no hesitation in seeking care. On the other hand, they may be less willing to do so for more sensitive matters. For example, a young woman may prefer to turn to her mother for advice and help, rather than to a nurse or a doctor when she suffers from painful menstrual periods.

Not surprisingly, a key factor that influences adolescents' health care-seeking behaviour is whether or not the act of seeking health care could get them into trouble with their parents or guardians. If, as in many cultures, social norms strongly forbid premarital sex, unmarried adolescents are likely to be wary about seeking care even if they have a painful genital ulcer or a possible unwanted pregnancy. They are likely to try to deal with the problem themselves, or with the help of friends or siblings whom they can trust to keep their secrets. To ensure that no one around them comes to learn about their problem, they tend to turn to service delivery points such as pharmacies and clinics at a safe distance from their homes, as well as to service providers who are as keen as they are to maintain secrecy (such as those who carry out abortions illegally).

---

5 Patton GC, Coffey C, Sawyer SM et al. Global patterns of mortality in young people. A systematic analysis of population data. *The Lancet*, 2009, 374: 881–892.

6 Gore F, Bloem PJN, Patton GC et al. Global burden of disease in young people aged 10—24 years: a systematic analysis. *The Lancet*, 2011, 377: 2093–2102.

7 Barker G, Olukoya A and Aggleton P. Young people, social support and help-seeking. *International Journal of Adolescent Medical Health*, 2005, 17, 4:315–336.

In many instances it is the adults surrounding an adolescent who decide whether or not health care needs to be sought, and if so when and where it should be sought. This is generally true in case of younger adolescents who are dependent on their parents. In some places, this is also true in case of older adolescents. Studies in several south Asian countries suggest that decisions on care-seeking during pregnancy and at the time of delivery, rest with husbands and mothers-in-law, rather than with young wives.

What are the barriers that adolescents face in obtaining the health services they need?

Some of the barriers that adolescents face in obtaining the health services they need also affect children and adults; others are specific to adolescents. These barriers relate to the availability, accessibility, acceptability and equity of health services.[8]

Firstly, in many places, health services such as emergency contraception and safe abortion are simply *not available to anyone*, either to adolescents or to adults.

Secondly, even where health services are available, adolescents may be unable to obtain them for a variety of reasons – restrictive laws and policies may prevent some health services from being provided to some groups of adolescents (e.g. the provision of contraceptives to unmarried adolescents); adolescents may not know where and when health services are provided; health facilities may be located a long distance from where they live/study/work; or health services may be expensive and beyond their reach). What this means is that the health services are *not accessible* to them.

Thirdly, health services may be delivered in a way that adolescents do not want to obtain them, even if they can. One common reason for this is that they have to go to, and wait in, a place where they could be seen by people they know. Other reasons are the fear that health workers will scold them, ask them difficult questions, and put them through unpleasant procedures; or that health workers will not maintain confidentiality. What this means is that the health services are *not acceptable* to them.

Finally, health services may be 'friendly' to some adolescents, such as those from well-to-do families, but may be decidedly 'unfriendly' to others, such as young people living and working on the streets. In other words, they may be available, accessible and acceptable but not necessarily *equitable*.

What do adolescents perceive as 'friendly' health services?

Adolescents are a heterogeneous group. The expectations and preferences of different groups of adolescents are understandably different.

It is interesting to note, however, that different groups of adolescents, from various parts of the world, identify two key, common characteristics. They want to be treated with respect and to be sure that their confidentiality is protected.[9]

---

8 *Adolescent-friendly health services: An agenda for change.* Geneva, World Health Organization, 2003.

What is being done to make to make health services adolescent friendly?

There is growing recognition of the need to overcome these barriers and to make it easier for adolescents to obtain the health services they need. Initiatives are being undertaken in many countries to help ensure that:[9]

- Health service providers are non judgemental and considerate in their dealings with adolescents; and they have the competencies needed to deliver the right health services in the right way.
- Health facilities are equipped to provide adolescents with the health services they need; and are also appealing and 'friendly' to adolescents.
- Adolescents are aware of where they can obtain the health services they need, and are both able and willing to do so when needed.
- Community members are aware of the health-service needs of different groups of adolescents, and support their provision.

NGOs are in the forefront of these efforts in most places, although in a growing number of countries, government-run health facilities are also reorienting themselves in order to reach out to adolescents. Initiatives are being undertaken in a variety of settings:

- Hospitals;
- Public, private and NGO clinics;
- Pharmacies;
- Youth centres;
- Educational institutions;
- Work places;
- Shopping centres;
- Refugee camps;
- On the street.

Most of these initiatives are small in scale and of limited duration. However, there are a steadily growing number of initiatives that have moved beyond the 'pilot' or 'demonstration project' stage to scale up their operations to reach out to adolescents across an entire district, province or country.

Is there any evidence that efforts to make health services adolescent friendly can increase their utilization by adolescents?

There is growing evidence for the effectiveness of some of these initiatives in improving the way health services are provided, and in increasing their use by adolescents.

In 2006, WHO published a systematic review of the effectiveness of interventions to improve the use of health services by adolescents in developing countries.[10] This review identified twelve initiatives, including one randomized controlled trial (Nigeria), six quasi-experimental studies (Bangladesh, China, Madagascar, Mongolia, Uganda and Zimbabwe), two national programmes (Mozambique and South Africa), and three projects (Ghana, Rwanda and Zimbabwe), which demonstrated that actions to make health services user friendly and appealing had led to increases – sometimes substantial– in the use of health services by adolescents.

---

9 *Global Consultation on adolescent-friendly health services. A consensus statement.* Geneva, World Health Organization, 2002.

10 Dick B, Ferguson J, Chandra-Mouli V, Brabin L et al. A review of the evidence for interventions to increase young people's use of health services in developing countries in Ross D, Dick B, J Ferguson (Eds.). *Preventing HIV/AIDS in young people: A systematic review of the evidence from developing countries.* Geneva, World Health Organization, 2006.

These conclusions were reiterated in another review published in 2008, which concluded that: *"Enough is known that a priority for the future is to ensure that each country, state and locality has a policy and support to encourage provision of innovative and well-assessed youth-friendly health services."*[11]

What can be done to improve the quality of health service provision to adolescents?

The starting point for any initiative aimed at improving the quality of health service provision to adolescents is the national health policy and strategy developed by the ministry of health, which will provide answers to five critical questions:

- What health outcomes are being aimed for?
- Among which group (or groups) of adolescents are these health outcomes being aimed for?
- What is the place of health service provision to adolescents within an overall strategy to achieve these health outcomes?
- What is the package of health services to be provided, to achieve the health outcomes being aimed for?
- Where (which type of health facility) and by whom (which type of health service provider) should these health services be provided by?

Precise answers to these questions will provide a sound basis for developing a national strategy to improve the quality of health service provision to adolescents.

It is important to build on what already exists. What this means is that efforts should be directed at making existing service-delivery points – intended to provide health services to all segments of the population – more friendly to adolescents, rather than on setting up new service-delivery points exclusively intended for adolescents. Having said that, dedicated health service-delivery points and outreach work could play a useful role in reaching marginalized and stigmatized groups of adolescents (such as injection drug users), who may be reluctant to use a service-delivery point that is open to all.

Two complementary efforts are needed – firstly, to make health-service provision friendly, so that adolescents are more likely to be able and willing to obtain the health services they need; and secondly, to ensure that the health services that adolescents need to stay healthy or to get back to good health are in fact being provided, and are being provided in the right manner. In other words, efforts must be made to increase both health service utilization and health service provision.

The WHO 'quality of care' framework provides a useful guide to work on improving health service provision and utilization.[12] It brings together the complementary imperatives of, on the one hand, making it easier for adolescents to obtain the health services they need and, on the other, providing them with the health services they need in the right way.

The quality of care framework provides a useful working definition of adolescent-friendly health services. To be considered adolescent friendly, health services should be accessible, acceptable, equitable, appropriate and effective, as outlined below:[13]

Accessible

Adolescents *are able to* obtain the health services that are available.

---

11 Tylee A, Haller DM, Graham T, Churchill R et al Youth-friendly primary-care services: how are we doing and what more needs to be done. The Lancet, 2007, 369.
12 *Quality of Care. A process for making strategic choices in health systems.* Geneva, World Health Organization, 2006.
13 *Quality Assessment Guidebook. A guide to assessing health services for adolescent clients.* Geneva, World Health Organization, 2009.

Acceptable

Adolescents *are willing to* obtain the health services that are available.

Equitable

All adolescents, not just selected groups, are able to obtain the health services that are available.

Appropriate

The *right health services* (i.e. the ones they need) are provided to them

Effective

The *right health services are provided in the right way*, and make a positive contribution to their health.

It provides a useful way of organizing the characteristics that have been shown in research and in programmatic experience to contribute to making health services adolescent friendly (see also Annex 1).

Specifying standards, i.e. statements of required quality,[14] is a key first step. Once that is done actions need to be taken to achieve those standards. A standards-driven quality improvement approach enables this to be accomplished in the following three ways:

1. It helps set clear goals for different aspects of service-delivery point operations. For example, a standard statement could specify what medicines (e.g. antibiotics) and supplies (e.g. needles and syringes, cotton swabs and spirit to clean injection sites) need to be in place in a service-delivery point. It could also specify the quantity of each of these medicines and supplies that need to be in place.

2. It provides the basis for assessing the achievement of goals. In relation to the example, the standard statement provides a basis to assess whether in a particular service-delivery point, the specified medicines and supplies are in place, and whether the specified quantities of these medicines and supplies are in place.

3. It provides an entry point for identifying why the goals were not achieved.

Based on this standards can help indicate what needs to be done, by when and by whom for the goals to be achieved. In relation to the example, if antibiotics to treat sexually transmitted infections in adolescents and adults are out of stock, the main reasons for this and actions to solve the problem – and to prevent it from occurring again in the future – need to be identified. These actions may need to be taken at the point service delivery, or they may need to be taken at other levels, for example at the district or national level. Once these actions are put in place, the situation must be reviewed periodically to determine whether specific problems recur.

Using these three complementary aspects – defining quality, measuring quality and improving quality – ministries of health can put in place national initiatives to improve the quality of health service provision to adolescents in order to achieve clearly defined health outcomes.[15] This can be done as part of wider initiatives to improve the quality of health services intended for all segments of the population.

---

14 E Necohea, D Bossemeyer. *Standards based management and recognition. A practical approach for improving the performance and quality of health services.* Baltimore, Jhpiego, 2005.

15 R Massoud, K Askov, J Reinke et al. *A modern paradigm for improving health care quality.* Bethesda, Quality Assurance Project, 2001.

What can be done to ensure that high quality health services reach all the adolescents who need them?

Scaling up has been defined by WHO and ExpandNet as: *"Deliberate efforts to increase the impact of successfully tested health innovations so as to benefit more people and to foster policy and programme development on a lasting basis."*[16] Deliberate efforts are needed to reach out to all adolescents who need health services.

Using the WHO nine-step approach to developing a scaling up strategy,[17] a systematic process has been developed for scale-up of health service provision to adolescents. The process begins with actions at the national level, which are followed by subsequent actions at the state/district level and the health facility levels. The process is outlined in the document titled: Strengthening the health sector response to adolescent health and development.[18]

---

16 *Practical guidance on scaling up health service innovations.* Geneva, World Health Organization (with ExpandNet), 2009.
17 Nine steps to developing a scaling up strategy. Geneva, World Health Organization (with ExpandNet), 2010.
18 *Strengthening the health sector's response to adolescent health and development.* Geneva, World Health Organization, 2009.

CHAPTER 2

Section I. Develop a shared understanding of adolescent health and strengthening health service provision to adolescents

There is one step in this section:

1. Develop a clear understanding of WHO's approach to promoting adolescent health, and to providing adolescents with the health services they need, among key stakeholders involved in the national effort to strengthen health service provision to adolescents.

What is the step?

– Develop a clear understanding of the WHO approach to promoting adolescent health and to providing adolescents with the health services they need, among key stakeholders involved in the national effort to strengthen health service provision to adolescents.

What is the purpose of this step?

– To ensure that key stakeholders involved in the national effort to strengthen health service provision to adolescents have a clear understanding of WHO's approach to promoting adolescent health and to providing adolescents with the health services they need. Key stakeholders may include officials from the ministry of health, officials from influential national NGOs, academics, and representatives of international organizations.

What is the importance of this step?

– The overall initiative is much more likely to move ahead if the key stakeholders have a shared understanding of promoting adolescent health and of providing adolescents with the health services they need.

How could this step be taken?

– In both formal and informal meetings with individuals, small groups or large groups, seek to understand the perspectives of key stakeholders and to explain the WHO approach to promoting adolescent health and to providing adolescents with the health services they need. (Please refer to Chapter 1).

Section II. Establish the basis for formulating the national quality standards for health service provision to adolescents, in national HIV/AIDS and/or reproductive health policies and strategies*

There are two steps in this section:

1. Establish the basis for addressing adolescents within the national HIV/AIDS and/or reproductive health (RH) policies and strategies.
2. Establish the basis for the provision of health services to adolescents within the framework of the national HIV/AIDS and/or RH policies and strategies.

What is step 1?
- Establish the basis for addressing adolescents within the national HIV/AIDS and/or RH policies and strategies.

What is the purpose of this step?
- To establish that this initiative is in line with national policies and strategies.

What is the importance of taking this step?
- Firstly, in many countries there are individuals, groups and organizations who are uncomfortable with providing adolescents sexual and reproductive health information and services. If there is resistance to the initiative from any quarter, it would be helpful to show that it is entirely in line with national policies and strategies.
- Secondly, grounding the initiative in national policies and strategies may make it more likely that it will receive both moral and material support of decision-makers in the government and in international organizations.

How could this step be taken?
- Review the national HIV/AIDS and RH policy and strategy documents.
- Hold one-to-one/small group discussions with officials responsible for the national HIV/AIDS and RH programmes.
- Based on your findings, prepare a paper and table this for discussion in the process leading to the development of the national quality standards for health service provision to adolescents. Some suggested questions to ask include:
  (i) Does the national HIV/AIDS and/or RH policy/strategy identify adolescents as a population group to be addressed?
  (ii) Does the national HIV/AIDS or RH policy/strategy identify:- the magnitude of the problem(s) in adolescents (e.g. the prevalence of HIV infection in males aged 15–19 years among the general population);
- the behaviours that contribute to the problem(s) in adolescents, (e.g. the prevalence of unprotected sexual activity with multiple partners);
- the factors influencing these behaviours in adolescents (e.g. low perception of the risk of HIV)?
  (i) Does the national HIV/AIDS and/or RH policy/strategy include a component to prevent HIV/AIDS and RH problems in adolescents?

What is step 2?
- Establish the basis for the provision of health services to adolescents within the framework of the national HIV/AIDS and/or RH policies/strategies.

What is the purpose of this step?
- To ensure that the national quality standards for health service provision to adolescents are formulated in line with national policies and strategies.

What is the importance of taking this step?
- Grounding the initiative in national policies and strategies will make it more likely that it will receive both the moral and the material support of decision-makers in the government and in international organizations.

* Where national adolescent health policies and strategies address HIV and Sexual and Reproductive Health, they should be reviewed.

> How could this step be taken?
>
> - Review the national HIV/AIDS and RH policy and strategy documents.
> - Hold one to-one/small group discussions with officials responsible for national HIV/AIDS and reproductive health programmes.
> - Based on your findings, prepare a paper and table this for discussion in the consultancy process leading to the formulation of the national quality standards.
>
> To begin with, point to the sections of the national HIV/AIDS and/or reproductive health policies/strategies that identify the need to provide sexual and reproductive health services to adolescents? Then, move on the following points.
>
> (i) The population groups to be addressed.
>
> (Note: Do the policy/strategy documents specify whether the health outcomes are being aimed for in all adolescents or only in some groups of adolescents?).
>
> (ii) The health outcomes being aimed for.
>
> (Note: Do the policy/strategy documents specify what changes in the health status are being aimed for?).
>
> (iii) The role of health service provision within a broader strategy.
>
> (Note: Do the policy/strategy documents specify that health service provision is grounded in a broader strategy that includes providing information and education to adolescents, providing them with counselling services, and making their environment safer and more supportive?).
>
> (iv) The package of health services to be provided.
>
> (Note: Do the policy/strategy documents specify the package of preventive and curative health services that need to be delivered at the primary and at various referral levels in order to contribute to the desired health outcomes?).
>
> (v) The delivery of these health services – where and by whom.
>
> (Note: Do the policy/strategy documents specify where (i.e. from which health service delivery points) and by whom (i.e. which health-service providers) the stipulated package of health services should be delivered ?).
>
> (vi) A clear position on the authorization of adolescents to obtain the health services they need, and the requirement for the consent of parents/guardians.
>
> (*Note:* Do the policy/strategy documents clearly state whether all groups of adolescents are authorized to obtain the stipulated package of health services; and whether they can do so autonomously – i.e. without the consent of parents or guardians).

Section III. Examine the programmatic implications of applying the national quality standards

There are four steps in this section:

1. Develop a clear understanding of what a standards-driven initiative to improve the quality and expand the coverage of health service provision to adolescents means in practice, and what it takes to translate quality-standard statements into tangible improvements in quality and coverage at health service delivery points, among key stakeholders involved in the national effort to strengthen health service provision to adolescents.

2. Develop a good understanding of the current situation regarding the provision of health services to adolescents, and their utilization by adolescents.

3. Gather experiences from within the country in applying quality improvement principles and practices in public health programmes.

4. Identify the place of the unit driving of the national standards-driven initiative in the country; as well as programmatic opportunities and challenges in applying them.

What is step 1?
– Develop a clear understanding of what a standards-driven initiative to improve quality and expand the coverage of health service provision to adolescents means in practice, and what it takes to translate quality-standard statements into tangible improvements in quality and coverage at health service delivery points, among key stakeholders involved in the national effort to strengthen health service provision to adolescents.

What is the purpose of this step?
– To seek to learn/understand from stakeholders:
  (i) what problem do they want to solve and what gap do they want to fill through this national standards-driven initiative to improve quality and expand coverage;
  (ii) what results do they expect to achieve through this initiative.
– To ensure that the key stakeholders clearly understand:
  (i) what a standards-driven initiative to improve the quality and expand the coverage of health service provision means in practice;
  (ii) what efforts are required at the national and district levels to translate the quality standard statements into tangible improvements in the quality of health service provision at health service delivery points.

What is the importance of taking this step?
– It is important to ensure that the key stakeholders involved in the national effort to strengthen health service provision to adolescents have a clear and shared understanding of the issues listed above. It is important that they are fully aware that this effort requires concerted and complementary efforts at national, district and local levels.

How could this step be taken?
Through formal and informal meetings with individuals, small or large groups, seek to understand the perspectives of key stakeholders and to inform/explain to them WHO's viewpoints on this. Do this using the accompanying slide sets and talking points.

What is step 2?
– Develop a good understanding of the current situation regarding the provision of health services to adolescents, and their utilization by adolescents.

What is the purpose of this step?
– To understand the current situation regarding:
  (i) by whom – and where – health services are currently provided to adolescents;
  (ii) barriers to the provision and utilization of health services by adolescents;
  (iii) help-seeking and health care-seeking practices of adolescents;
  (iv) initiatives that are under way in providing adolescents with the health services they need.

What is the importance of this step?
Firstly, a good understanding of the current situation will provide a solid basis for considering how the situation could be improved, building on the areas of strength, and addressing gaps and areas of weakness. Secondly, it will send a clear message that there is a systematic effort to draw upon, the lessons learned from within the country, in this area.

How could this step be taken?
– Through discussions with key informants in the ministry of health, NGOs, academic institutions and international agencies, gather published papers and reports on:
  (i) by whom – and where – health services are currently provided to adolescents;
  (ii) barriers to the provision and utilization of health services by adolescents;
  (iii) help-seeking and health care-seeking practices of adolescents;
  (iv) initiatives that are under way in providing adolescents with the health services they need.
(Note: It is important to obtain the view points and perspectives of different groups of adolescents).
– Identify individuals and organizations that are carrying out research and/or implementing programmes/projects on health service provision to adolescents.

– If possible, bring together a small working group to prepare a working paper highlighting the lessons that could be drawn from their work for scaling up health service provision to adolescents.
– Identify possible individuals who could be involved in the formulation of the national quality standards

What is step 3?
- Gather experiences from within the country in applying quality improvement principles and practices in public health programmes.

What is the purpose of this step?
- To draw out the experiences gained from initiatives in the country that have worked to improve the quality of health service provision and to increase health service utilization by any population group in order to achieve a clearly defined health outcome.

What is the importance of taking this step?
- There are three potential benefits of doing this. Firstly, it will help communicate the message that quality improvement principles and practices are not foreign to the country. Secondly, it will help key stakeholders to understand what the application of quality improvement principles and practices can achieve, and more importantly what it takes to put and keep them in place. Thirdly, it will point to individuals and organizations from within the country whose expertise could be drawn upon.

How could this step be taken?
- Through discussions with key informants in the ministry of health, NGOs, academic institutions and international agencies, identify noteworthy initiatives that have applied quality improvement principles and practices in public health work.
- Gather published papers or reports that describe the process employed by these initiatives and the results they achieved.
- Identify individuals and organizations that are carrying out research and/or implementing programmes/projects on health service provision to adolescents.
- If possible, bring together a small working group to prepare a working paper highlighting the lessons that could be drawn from their work for scaling up health service provision to adolescents.

What is step 4?
- Identify the place of the unit driving the national standards-driven initiative in the country; as well as programmatic opportunities and challenges in applying them.

What is the purpose of this step?
- To identify the 'driver' of the national standards-driven initiative, the strengths and weaknesses of the unit, and its linkages with other units in the ministry of health.
- To identify factors in the environment that could help or hinder the implementation of the initiative. For example, a national effort to improve the quality of reproductive health services supported by UNFPA could be a potential opportunity for a link with the initiative. However, the lack of willingness to engage health-service providers in the private sector in public health programmes could hinder the ability of the initiative to work with a key group who many groups of adolescents turn to.

What is the importance of taking this step?
- Firstly, the national standards-driven initiative to improve the quality and expand the coverage of health service provision to adolescents is much more likely to succeed if it has a driver with the authority, the technical capacity and the resources needed to move the initiative forward.
- Secondly, in moving the initiative forward it is important to be aware of potential opportunities and challenges in the environment.

How could this step be taken?
- Through discussions with key informants in the ministry of health, NGOs, academic institutions and international agencies, identify programmatic openings, prepare a working paper on:
    (i) what are the strengths and weaknesses of the driver of the initiative, and what could be done to build on the strengths and address the weaknesses;
    (ii) the potential opportunities and challenges in implementing the initiative.

Section IV. Develop the national standards

There are two steps in this section:

1. Obtain the public support of the key stakeholders whose support is important for the national standards-driven quality improvement to succeed.
2. Develop the national standards (and accompanying elements of a standards-driven quality improvement initiative).

What is step 1?
- Obtain the support of a wide range of stakeholders whose support is important for the national standards-driven quality improvement initiative to succeed. In addition to individuals and organizations involved in the preparatory work, this step should involve other community members such as political leaders, religious leaders, teachers and officials from government departments other than health whose work affects adolescents/young people. It is important to involve adolescents as well in the consultative process.

What is the purpose of this step?
- To present the conclusions and recommendations of the preparatory work that has been done (as described in sections I, II and III) and to obtain further inputs.
- To place in the public arena the fact that the national standards are to be developed and the ground work that has been done to prepare for this.

What is the importance of taking this step?
- For the initiative to succeed it is important to ensure that the wide range of stakeholders referred to above are fully aware that national standards for health service provision to adolescents are being developed and comfortable with the process for this. Secondly, they must be fully aware of the preparatory work that has been done and satisfied that it is adequate. Thirdly, they need to believe that their perspectives have been listened to and taken on board.

How could this step be taken?
- Organize a consensus-building workshop bringing together a wide range of stakeholders.

(Note: It is important to involve adolescents in the consultative process. This could be done by having one or more meetings in advance of the national consensus-building workshop. Adolescents selected by their peers could be invited to participate in the consensus-building workshop.

What is step 2?
- Develop the national standards (and accompanying elements of a standards-driven quality improvement initiative).

What is the purpose of this step?
- To define the key problems (i.e. the gap between required quality and actual quality) that the standards seek to address.
- For each problem:
  (i) To formulate the standards (i.e. the desired quality to be achieved),
  (ii) To identify the input, process and output criteria to achieve each standard (i.e. what needs to in place and what needs to happen in and around at points of health service delivery for the standard to be achieved),
  (iii) To identify the actions needed at national, district and local level to achieve each criteria,
  (iv) To identify the indicators to verify the achievement of the criteria, and means of verifying them.

What is the importance of taking this step?
- This step clearly outlines the objectives of the national initiative seeks to achieve, what needs to be done to achieve these objectives, and what needs to be done to assess whether these objectives are being achieved.

> How could this step be taken?
> - A working group consisting of 8–10 persons should work together to draft the standards. Here is an indicative list of working group members:
>   (i) 1–2 officials from the ministry of health at the national level;
>   (ii) 1–2 persons from influential NGOs;
>   (iii) 1–2 academics;
>   (iv) 1–2 representatives of international organizations.
> - The draft standards should be shared with key stakeholders involved in the national effort to strengthen health service provision to adolescents.
> - The working group should meet, possibly more than once, to review the feedback that has been received, and work to revise and finalize the standards.
>
> (*Note:* The accompanying presentation entitled *Developing standards* and the accompanying document titled *Generic characteristics of adolescent-friendly health services within WHO-defined dimensions of quality*, can be used to guide the development of the standards and other elements).

Section V. Outline essential preparatory work at national levels before the quality standards can be applied

There are four steps in this section:

1. Ensure that the draft standards and accompanying elements, are cleared by the relevant authorities after being reviewed and revised, as needed.

2. Develop an implementation guide that outlines what district health management teams and managers of health facilities need to do to ensure that the structure criteria accompanying each standard statement are in place.

3. Develop a monitoring guide that outlines what and how district health management teams and managers of health facilities need to track implementation.

4. Inform key stakeholders at the national level, who could help or hinder the implementation of the initiative; explain to them what it aims to achieve and how it aims to do this.

> **What is step 1?**
> - Ensure that the draft standards and accompanying elements are cleared by the relevant authorities after being reviewed and revised, as needed.

> What is the purpose of this step?
> - To have the standards and accompanying endorsed by the relevant authorities, and thereby translating them into an authoritative national document.

> What is the importance of taking this step?
> - Official endorsement is required before the document can be disseminated and applied in order to improve the quality of health services.

> How could this step be taken?
> - Actively follow up with the relevant authorities for official clearance. This will require responding to questions and clarifying any lingering misconceptions.

> **What is step 2?**
> - Develop an implementation guide that outlines what district health management teams and managers of health facilities need to do to ensure that the structure criteria accompanying each standard statement are in place.

What is the purpose of this step?
- To provide clear guidance to district health management teams and managers of health facilities on what they need to do to ensure that the \structure criteria accompanying each standard are put in place.

What is the importance of taking this step?
- It is important to ensure that district health management teams and managers of heath facilities are clear as to what they need to do to ensure that the structure criteria accompanying each standard are put in place. Without clear guidance, it is likely that essential things may not be done.

How could this step be taken?
- Identify and engage an individual/organization with expertise in this area to prepare an implementation guide. For example, structure criteria 4 (which accompanies standard 2 in the Tanzanian standards for youth-friendly reproductive health services) states: "Equipment, supplies and medicines will be constantly available". In this case, the implementation guide needs to specify the range – and quantities – of equipment, supplies and medicines that need to be place in each health facility.

What is step 3?
- Develop a monitoring guide that outlines what and how district health management teams and managers of health facilities need to track implementation.

What is the purpose of this step?
- To provide clear guidance to district health management teams and managers of health facilities on what and how they need to check in order to verify that the required actions are being carried out.

What is the importance of taking this step?
- It is important for district health management teams and managers of health facilities to be clear about what exactly they need to check and how they should do this.

How could this step be taken?
- Identify and engage an individual/organization with the expertise in this area, to prepare a monitoring guide.

What is step 4?
- Inform key stakeholders at the national level, who could help or hinder the implementation of the initiative; explain to them what it aims to achieve and how it aims to do this.

What is the purpose of this step?
- To ensure that stakeholders do not oppose the initiative, and where relevant to draw upon their support in moving forward.

What is the importance of taking this step?
- Firstly, key stakeholders may have the power to 'kill' the initiative themselves. Alternatively, they could contribute to its decline by speaking about it in a negative manner. They may do this because they do not understand fully, because they believe – or may hear – that it is not useful/feasible, or because they may feel excluded from the consultative process contributing to the initiative. Secondly, they may be able to provide useful ideas and suggestions to strengthen the initiative. Thirdly, they may be willing and able to support the initiative.

How could this step be taken?
- Identify the key stakeholders who need to be reached. Here is an indicative list:
  (i) Within the ministry of health: the national HIV/AIDS programme, the national reproductive health programme, and the primary health care unit;
  (ii) The ministry of local government;
  (iii) Key international organizations: within the United Nations system, bilateral agencies, international organizations;
  (iv) National NGOs.
- Ideally, set up one-to-one meetings to explain the initiative, request ideas and suggestions for moving it forward.
- Use an appropriate forum, such as a regular meetings of the national HIV/AIDS programme, to inform them about the initiative and obtain their support for it.

CHAPTER 3

This chapter contains materials that can be used to prepare and conduct a workshop to develop national quality standards for adolescent-friendly health services.

Outline of the background paper for a national workshop to develop national quality standards on adolescent-friendly health services

Aim of the paper:

a. To establish the basis for the provision of health services to adolescents within the framework of the national policies and strategies on adolescent health, reproductive health or HIV.

b. To develop a good understanding of the current situation regarding the provision of health services to adolescents, and their utilization by adolescents.

Outline of content:

Part 1 Analysis of existing policies/strategies

1. The health outcomes being aimed for.

(*Note:* Do the policy/strategy documents specify what changes in the health status are being aimed for?).

2. The population groups to be addressed.

(*Note:* Do the policy/strategy documents specify whether the these health outcomes are being aimed for in all adolescents or in some groups of adolescents?).

3. The role of health service provision within a broader strategy.

(*Note:* Do the policy/strategy documents specify that health service provision is grounded in a broader strategy, which includes providing information and education to adolescents, providing them with counselling services, and making their environment safer and more supportive?).

4. The package of health services to be provided.

(Note: Do the policy/strategy documents specify the package of preventive and curative health services that need to be delivered at the primary and at the referral levels to contribute to the desired health outcomes?).

5. The delivery of these health services – where and by whom?

(Note: Do the policy/strategy documents specify where (i.e. from which health service delivery points) and by whom (i.e. which health service providers) the stipulated package of health services should be delivered?).

6. A clear position on the authorization of adolescents to obtain the health services they need, and the requirement for the consent of parents/guardians.

(Note: Do the policy/strategy documents clearly state whether all groups of adolescents are authorized to obtain the stipulated package of health services?).

Part 2 Current situation regarding the provision to and use of health services by adolescents

For a good understanding of the current situation regarding the provision of health services to adolescents, and their utilization, gather information on the following issues:

1. The current situation in terms of health service provision to adolescents and their utilization by them. By whom – and where – are health services currently being provided to adolescents. Initiatives that are under way in providing adolescents with the health services they need. (Note: It is very important to obtain the viewpoints and perspectives of different groups of adolescents).
2. Barriers to the provision to and utilization of health services by adolescents.
3. Help-seeking, and health care-seeking practices of adolescents.
4. Individuals and organizations that are carrying out research and/or implementing programmes/projects on health service provision to adolescents.
5. The lessons that could be drawn from their work for scaling up health service provision to adolescents.

Part 3 National experiences in applying quality improvement and coverage expansion principles and practices in public health, even if this does not address adolescents

1. Brief descriptions of noteworthy initiatives that have applied quality improvement principles and practices in public health work.
2. A list of published papers or reports that describe the process employed by these initiatives and the results that they achieved.
3. A list of individuals and organizations that are carrying out research and/or implementing programmes/projects on quality control of health services, even if not addressed directly to adolescents.
4. Lessons that could be drawn from items 1–3 above for application in developing national quality standards for adolescent-friendly health services
5. Opportunities and challenges in setting up a national quality improvement and coverage expansion initiative to strengthen health service provision to adolescents.

Workshop to develop national quality standards for adolescent-friendly health services: Objectives, agenda and facilitators guide

Objectives

To draft national quality standards and accompanying elements for providing health services to adolescents.

Agenda

Days	9.00 to 10.30	11.00 to 12.30	14.00 to 15.30	16.00 to 17.30
1	– Opening remarks – Introductions – Statement of objectives of the workshop – Explanation of working methods to be used	– Identify the intended beneficiaries	– Define the health outcomes to be achieved	– Define the health services and health-related commodities to be delivered
2	– Identify the health service and health-related commodity delivery points	– Identify the problem statements to be addressed	– Formulate the quality standards	
3	– Choose the set of criteria to be achieved for each quality standard to be achieved		– Identify the actions to be taken at national, district and local levels for the criteria to be achieved	
4	– Specify ways and means of verifying the achievement of the criteria		– Outline the preparatory work that needs to be done at the national level before the quality standards can be applied	– Closing remarks

Facilitators guide for sessions

1. Identify the intended beneficiaries

Ask the following questions:

a. What is the population segment (e.g. 10–19 years) we want to address? Why?

b. Within this, which population group do we want to focus on? (E.g. those living and working on the street). Why?

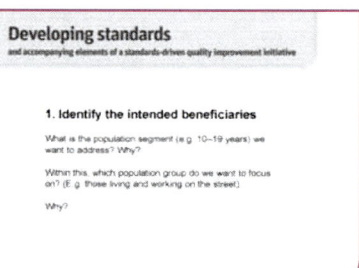

Tips for the facilitator

Deal with the first question in plenary. Ask the group to name the population segment to be addressed and the rationale for this.

For the second question, split up the larger group into 'buzz groups' of 3 people. Ask each group to identify a maximum of two population groups and to provide the rationale for their choice. Ask each buzz group to share their conclusions in plenary. Work with them to arrive at a list of around 5 specific population groups.

2. Define the health outcomes to be achieved

Ask the following question:

2.1 What are the health outcomes we want to achieve? Why?

Tips for the facilitator

Prepare copies of the following table in advance of the workshop.

Split up the larger group into buzz groups of 3 people. Ask each group to fill in the table. When they are done, ask them to share their outputs in plenary. Work with them to arrive at a short list of health outcomes to be addressed, using the criteria listed in the table. Stress that the longer the list is, the more challenging this will be for implementation.

Health outcomes	How relevant is this issue in my country? (1–5)	Can health workers make a meaningful contribution to addressing it? (1–5)
(i) Healthy development:		
To promote healthy development		
To respond to development problems when they occur		
(ii) Healthy nutrition:		
To prevent under- and over-nutrition		
To respond to under- and over-nutrition when they occur		
(iii) Sexual and reproductive health:		
To prevent unwanted pregnancy		
To respond to unwanted pregnancy when it occurs		
To support healthy pregnancy and to prevent problems during pregnancy		
To respond to problems when they occur during pregnancy		
To prevent sexually transmitted infections (STI)		
To respond to STI when they occur		
To prevent HIV infection		
To respond to HIV infection/HIV-related illnesses when they occur		
To prevent sexual violence		

Health outcomes	How relevant is this issue in my country? (1–5)	Can health workers make a meaningful contribution to addressing it? (1–5)
To respond to sexual violence when it occurs		
(iv) Mental health:		
To prevent mental health problems		
To respond to mental health problems when they occur		
(v) Substance use:		
To prevent substance use		
To respond to substance use problems when they occur		
(vi) Injuries:		
To prevent unintentional injuries		
To respond to the physical and psychological consequences of unintentional injuries when they occur		
(vii) Injuries resulting from violence:		
To prevent violence		
To respond to the physical and psychological consequences of violence when it occurs		
(viii) Endemic diseases:		
To prevent endemic diseases, such as malaria and dengue		
To respond to them when they occur		
(ix) Chronic conditions:		
To respond to chronic conditions when they occur		

3. Define the health services and commodities to be delivered to achieve these health outcomes

Ask the following question:

3.1 What are the health services to be provided in relation to each of the health outcomes above?

Tips for the facilitator

Depending on the size of the group, split them up into buzz groups of 3 people. Ask each group to address some of the health outcomes. Ask them to share their outputs in plenary. Based on the discussion revise and finalize the following table.

Health outcome to be achieved	Information provision	Counselling provision	Clinical service (promotive, preventive or curative)	Referral

4. Identify the health service and commodity deliver points

Ask the following questions:

4.1 Where are the health services to be provided?

4.2 Where are the health-related commodities to be provided?

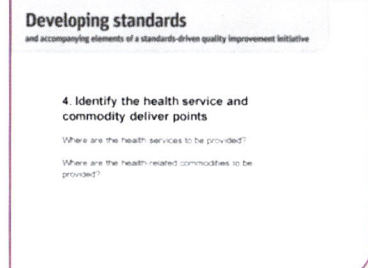

Tips for the facilitator

Depending on the size of the group, split them up into buzz groups of 3 people. Ask each group to address 1–2 delivery points, using the matrix below. Ask them to share their conclusions in plenary. Based on the discussion, finalize the matrix below.

Health service/ health-related commodity delivery points	Groups of adolescents who are likely to come in or to be reached	The health services that could be provided: - Information provision; - Counselling provision; - Clinical service provision; - Referral.	The health-related commodities that could be provided
A.			
B.			
C.			
D.			
E.			

5. Identify the problem statements (the gap between desired quality and actual quality)

Ask the following question:

How does each of the health service delivery points/health-related commodity delivery points relate to the desired quality?

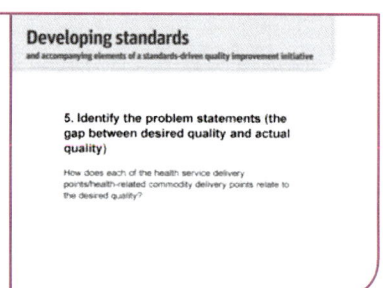

Task:

Identify key problems in the health service delivery points.

Tips for the facilitator

Do this exercise with the entire group. Ask participants to work together to complete the following matrix. Once all the problem statements are noted, ask the group to identify the five most important ones (using the following two criteria):

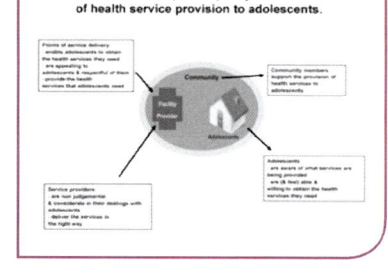

a. the size of the gap between the actual and desired quality;

b. which of the gaps are most relevant to the groups of adolescents we are concerned about?

Desired quality	Actual quality
Points of health service or health-related commodity delivery: – provide the health services and the health-related commodities that adolescents need (either-on the-spot or through referral linkages) – enable adolescents to obtain the health services they need – are appealing to adolescents	
Health workers: – are non-judgemental and considerate in their dealings with adolescents – deliver the services in the 'right' way	
Support staff: – are non-judgemental and considerate in their dealings with adolescents	
Community members support the provision of health services to adolescents	
Adolescents – are aware of what services are being provided – are (and feel) able and willing to obtain the health services they need.	

6. Formulate the quality standard statements

Ask the following question:

When we say that we want to improve the quality of these health service delivery points, what exactly do we mean?

Task:

Formulate standard statements in relation to each of the main problems identified. For each standard statement, define key words and phrases in the statement.

Tips for the facilitator

Explain to the group that a standard is defined as a statement of required quality. In other words, it is a precise description of what the situation will be like after the problem has been tackled and successfully addressed.

7. Choose the set of criteria to be achieved for each quality standard to be achieved

Ask the following question:

What needs to be in place for the quality standard to be achieved?

Task:

Choose the criteria needed to achieve each standard. In other words, identify what needs to be in place for each standard to be achieved.

Tips for the facilitator

Lead the group through an example. In doing so, explain to the group that there are three types of criteria:

   i. Input criteria: The 'hardware' that needs to be in place at a health service-delivery point

Examples: A competent health worker; a notice board listing the opening hours of a clinic.

   ii. Process criteria: The way in which staff in the health service delivery point deal with adolescent patients and with other community members.

Examples: Health workers manage adolescents as stated in the guidelines; support staff are welcoming to adolescents.

   iii. Output criteria: The desired effect on adolescent users of the health service delivery point and on other community members.

Examples: Adolescents feel that health workers are concerned about their welfare; community members are aware of what health services are being provided by the clinic.

Ask the group to brainstorm on possible criteria. Once this done, work with them to choose a short list based on the following issues:

- Potential impact (i.e. the potential impact of the criteria in contributing to the standard).
- Feasibility (i.e. the feasibility of putting the criteria in place, in the local context).
- Complementarity (i.e. how the set of criteria complement each other).

Stress that the criteria that they choose need to be ambitious but not overambitious, in line with national laws and policies, and sensitive to the social and cultural norms.

Standard statement # 1

Criteria					
Input criteria	Process criteria (that correspond to the input criteria)	Output criteria	Potential impact	Feasibility	Complementarity
1.					
2.					
3.					
4.					
5.					

8. Identify the actions to be taken at national, district and local levels for the criteria to be achieved

Ask the following question:

What needs to be done at the national, district and local levels to ensure that health service provision meets the specified quality?

Task:

Identify the actions that need to be taken to achieve each of the input criteria at the national, district and local levels.

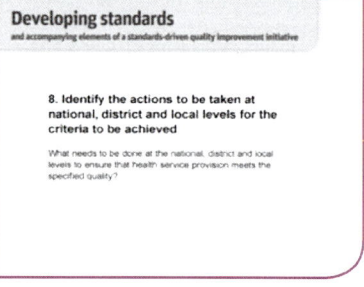

Tips for the facilitator

Lead the group through an example. In doing so, explain to the group that they need to identify actions that are required at the national, district and local levels. Stress that they need to consider the *complementary nature of these actions*. For example, a logo for the initiative will need to developed at the national level; officials at the district level will need to provide support to clinics in painting the logo on their notice boards; and clinic managers will need to ensure that their notice boards are not covered by unauthorised posters.

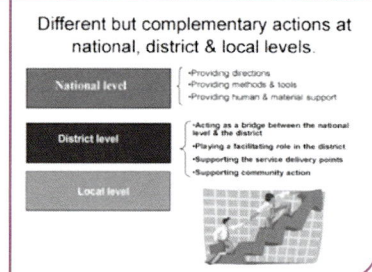

The actions that they identify – just like the criteria they have chosen – need to be:

- ambitious but not overambitious;
- in line with national laws and policies;
- sensitive to the social and cultural norms.

Please note that they only need to identify actions for the input criteria.

Standard statement # 1

Criteria				
Input criteria	Process criteria (that correspond to the input criteria)	Local level (i.e. health service delivery point)	District level	National level
1.				
2.				
3.				
4.				
5.				

9. Specify ways and means to verify the achievement of the criteria

Ask the following question:

How will we know that the elements contributing to the quality of health service provision are in place?

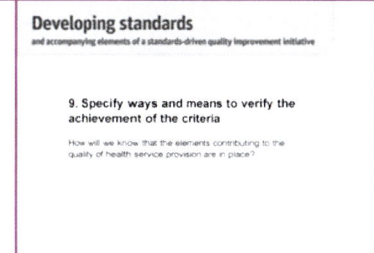

Task:

For each criteria specify:

- What data to gather in order to verify whether the criteria has been achieved;
- How to gather this data.

Tips for the facilitator

Lead the group through an example. In doing so, stress to the working group that for each item in the list they need to consider the *effort and the expense* of the proposed actions. Encourage them to use existing monitoring mechanisms as far as possible to reduce the cost and to increase the likelihood that monitoring will in fact be done.

Note that this will need to be done for input, process and output criteria.

Standard statement # 1

Criteria	What to verify?	How to verify?
Input criteria		
1.		
2.		
3.		
4.		
5.		
Process criteria:		
1.		
2.		
Output criteria:		
1.		
2.		

10. Outline the preparatory work that needs to be done at the national level before the quality standards can be applied

Ask the following question:

What groundwork needs to be done in order for all these ideas can be translated into reality?

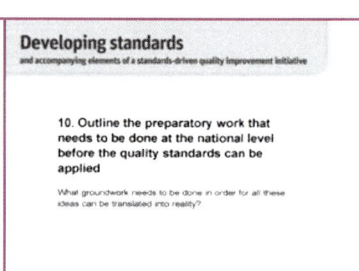

Task:

List the preparatory work that needs to be done before implementation can begin.

Tips for the facilitator

Do this exercise in plenary. Lead the group through a quick brainstorming session on what preparatory work needs to be done. Once you have a 6–8 points on a flip chart, ask them to review each item and to identify why it is important to do, using the following matrix:

What preparatory work needs to be done?	Why is this important?
1.	
2.	
3.	
4.	
5.	
6.	

7.	
8.	
9.	
10.	

Once the list has been completed, press the group to specify who will be responsible for each item and to propose a date by when the task has to be carried out.

What preparatory work needs to be done?	Who will be responsible for carrying out this task?	When will this task be carried out?
1.		
2.		
3.		
4.		
5.		
6.		
7.		
8.		
9.		
10.		

ANNEX 1

Generic characteristics of adolescent-friendly health services within WHO-defined dimensions of quality

Dimensions of quality health services to adolescents

Equitable
All adolescents, not just some groups of adolescents, are able to obtain the health services that are available.

Accessible
Adolescents *are able to* obtain the health services that are available.

Acceptable
Adolescents *are willing to* obtain the health services that are available.

Appropriate
The *right health services (i.e. the ones they need)* are provided to them.

Effective
The *right health services are provided in the right way*, and make a positive contribution to their health.

EQUITABLE: *All adolescents, not just some groups of adolescents*, are able to obtain the health services that are available
Characteristics
Policies and procedures are in place that do not restrict the provision of health services.
Health care providers treat all adolescent clients with equal care and respect, regardless of status.
Support staff treat all adolescent clients with equal care and respect, regardless of status.
ACCESSIBLE: Adolescents *are able to* obtain the health services that are available
Characteristics
Policies and procedures are in place that ensure that health services are either free or affordable to adolescents.
Point of service delivery has convenient working hours.
Adolescents are well informed about the range of reproductive health services available and how to obtain them.
Community members understand the benefits that adolescents will gain by obtaining the health services they need, and support their provision.
Some health services and health-related commodities are provided to adolescents in the community by selected community members, outreach workers and adolescents themselves.
ACCEPTABLE: Adolescents *are willing to* obtain the health services that are available
Characteristics
Policies and procedures are in place that guarantee client confidentiality.
Point of service delivery ensures privacy.
Health care providers are non-judgmental, considerate, and easy to relate to.
Point of service delivery ensures consultations occur in a short waiting time, with or without an appointment, and (where necessary) swift referral.
Point of service delivery has an appealing and clean environment.
Point of service delivery provides information and education through a variety of channels.
Adolescents are actively involved in designing, assessing and providing health services.
APPROPRIATE: he *right health services (i.e. the ones they need)* are provided to them
Characteristics
The required package of health care is provided to fulfil the needs of all adolescents either at the point of service delivery or through referral linkages.
EFFECTIVE: The *right health services are provided in the right way*, and make a positive contribution to their health
Characteristics
Health care providers have the required competencies to work with adolescents and to provide them with the required health services.
Health care providers use evidenced-based protocols and guidelines to provide health services.
Health care providers are able to dedicate sufficient time to deal effectively with their adolescent clients.
The point of service delivery has the required equipment, supplies, and basic services necessary to deliver the required health services.

To improve the equity of services at the point of delivery:

1. Policies and procedures are in place to ensure that the provision of health services is not restricted on any terms

(i) What does this mean?

There are no laws and policies that restrict the provision of health services by age, sex or any other area of difference.

Why is this important?

In many countries, as a result of existing laws and policies, the provision of some health services to all or some groups of adolescents is unauthorized or even illegal. These restrictive laws and policies are a serious obstacle to public health. They are also contrary to the *United Nations Convention on the Rights of the Child* that says that young people have a right to life, development, and "the highest attainable standard of health and to facilities for the treatment of illness and rehabilitation of health." (Article 24).

(ii) What does this mean?

Procedures are in place to ensure that no factor whether it be based on age, sex, social status, cultural background, ethnic origin, disability or any other reason:

- hinders the ***provision*** of health services to all or some groups of adolescents;
- hinders the ***ability*** of all or some adolescents from obtaining health services.

Why is this important?

In many places, existing procedures hinder the equitable provision of health services, and also of adolescents' experiences in obtaining them. Adolescents will not attend a point of service delivery if they feel excluded or discriminated against in any way.

2. Health care providers treat all their adolescent patients with equal care and respect, regardless of status

What does this mean?

Health care providers administer the same level of care and consideration to all adolescents regardless of age, sex, social status, cultural background, ethnic origin, disability or any other reason.

Why is this important?

Being treated disrespectfully is a strong disincentive for adolescents to seek help. Being treated equally will have a positive effect on adolescents, encouraging them to attend further appointments and recommend the service to their peers.

3. Support staff treat all their adolescent patients with equal care and respect, regardless of status

What does this mean?

Support staff administer the same level of care and consideration to all adolescents regardless of age, sex, social status, cultural background, ethnic origin, disability or any other reason.

Why is this important?

Being treated disrespectfully is a strong disincentive for adolescents to seek help. Being treated equally will have a positive effect on adolescents, encouraging them to attend further appointments and recommend the service to their peers.

To improve the accessibility of services at point of health service delivery

4. Policies and procedures are in place to ensure that health services are either free or affordable to all adolescents

What does this mean?

All adolescents are able to receive health services free of charge or are able to afford any charges that might be in place.

Why is this important?

This is particularly relevant in adolescents who are likely to have limited financial means of their own. Adolescents who are dependent on their families may not want to 'add to the burden' by asking for money to pay for services. They may also be reluctant to disclose why they need to obtain health services.

5. The point of health service delivery has convenient working hours

What does this mean?

Health services are available to all adolescents during times of the day that are convenient to them.

Why is this important?

Adolescents may find it difficult to obtain health services if the working hours coincide with times when they are busy with study, work or other activities.

6. Adolescents are well informed about the range of health services available and how to obtain them

What does this mean?

Adolescents are aware of what health services are being provided, where they are provided, and how to obtain them.

Why is this important?

Informing adolescents about the range of health services available to them can help to encourage usage of services.

7. Community members understand the benefits that adolescents will gain by obtaining health services, and support their provision

What does this mean?

Community members (including parents) are well informed about how the provision of health services could help their adolescents. They support the provision of these services as well as their use by adolescents.

Why is this important?

Communities are likely to oppose the provision of health services to adolescents if they do not understand – or trust – their value. Engaging community members in a respectful discussion and working to create a shared understanding on this issue will help to ensure that the required health services can be provided, and obtained, without opposition.

8. **Some health services and health-related supplies are provided to adolescents in the community by selected community members, by outreach workers and by adolescents themselves**

    What does this mean?

    Efforts are under way to provide health services close to where adolescents are. Depending on the situation, outreach workers, selected community members (e.g. sports coaches) and adolescents themselves may be involved in this.

    Why is this important?

    Adolescents may be reluctant to visit health facilities and other points of delivery. Some of them may be unable to do so. Outreach workers, selected community members and adolescents themselves can extend the reach of health services into the community. The provision of health information and services by people they can easily relate to and in places they frequent may be welcomed by adolescents.

To improve the acceptability of services at point of health service delivery level

9. **Policies and procedures are in place that guarantee client confidentiality**

    What does this mean?

    Policies and procedures are in place that maintain adolescent confidentiality at all times (except where staff are obliged by legal requirements to report incidents such as sexual assaults, road traffic accidents or gunshot wounds, to the relevant authorities).

    Policies and procedures address:

    - registration – information on the identify of the adolescent and the presenting issue are gathered in confidence;
    - consultation – confidentiality is maintained throughout the visit of the adolescent to the point of delivery (i.e. before, during and after a consultation);
    - record-keeping – case records are kept in a secure place, accessible only to authorized personnel;
    - disclosure of information – staff do not disclose any information given to or received from an adolescent, to a third party (for example, family members, school teachers or employers) without their consent.

    Why is this important?

    Adolescents are very sensitive to privacy and confidentiality. Adolescents from around the world say that concerns about lack of privacy and confidentiality discourage their use of health services.

10. The point of health service delivery ensures privacy

What does this mean?

The point of service delivery is located in a place that ensures the privacy of adolescent users. It has a layout that is designed to ensure privacy throughout an adolescent's visit. This includes the point of entry, the reception area, the waiting area, the examination area and the patient-record storage area.

Why is this important?

Adolescents give high priority to privacy. They are more likely to obtain the health services they need if they are confident that they will not be seen by anyone else, and that the privacy of their records will be maintained.

11. Health care providers are non-judgemental, considerate and easy to relate to

What does this mean?

Health care providers do not criticize their adolescent patients even if they do not approve of their words and actions. They are considerate to their patients and reach out to them in a friendly manner.

Why is this important?

Health care providers do not need to abandon their own beliefs and values, but they must ensure that these beliefs and values do not negatively influence the way in which they deal with their adolescent patients. In addition, the ability to respond to adolescents with empathy and sensitivity will contribute to the development of good communication and mutual respect.

Judgemental, inconsiderate and unfriendly behaviour will hinder communication. It is also likely to turn adolescents away.

12. The point of health service delivery ensures consultations occur in a short waiting time, with or without an appointment and (where necessary) swift referral

What does this mean?

Adolescents are able to consult with health care providers at short notice, whether they have a formal appointment or not. If their medical condition is such that they need to be referred elsewhere, the referral appointment should also take place within a short timeframe.

Why is this important?

Adolescents are more likely than adults to be deterred by long waiting times or by rigid appointment-making policies. Having to wait for an appointment in advance could lead to a missed appointment or seeking help from other possibly less effective or even harmful service providers offering shorter waiting times.

13. The point of health service delivery has an appealing and clean environment

What does this mean?

A point of health service delivery that is welcoming, attractive and clean.

Why is this important?

Adolescents – like adults – may not want to go to a poorly maintained and dirty place.

14. The point of health service delivery provides information using a variety of methods

What does this mean?

Informational materials that are relevant to the health of adolescents provided by the point of health service delivery are available in different formats (e.g. posters, booklets and leaflets). They are presented in a familiar language, are easy to understand and are eye-catching.

Why is this important?

Adolescents who visit the place may not know what they need to understand about the health problems that could affect them. They may have received incorrect information from their peers or other sources. They may have questions but may be embarrassed to ask their parents, teachers or others.

15. Adolescents are actively involved in the assessment and provision of health services

What does this mean?

Adolescents are given the opportunity to share their experiences in obtaining health services, and to express their needs and preferences. They are involved in certain appropriate aspects of health service provision.

Why is this important?

Involving adolescents in assessing service provision, and in actually participating in service provision, can help make health services more sensitive and responsive to their needs.

The appropriateness of health services for adolescents is best achieved if:

16. The health services required to fulfil the needs of all adolescents are provided either at the point of delivery or through referral linkages

What does this mean?

The health needs and problems of all adolescents are addressed by the health services provided at the point of health service delivery, or through referral linkages. The services provided meet the special needs of marginalized groups of adolescents, as well as those of the majority.

Why is this important?

All adolescents should be able to obtain the health services that meet their needs either from one point of health service delivery, or from a set of points that are linked together in a helpful manner.

The effectiveness of health services for adolescents is best achieved if:

17. Health care providers have the required competencies

What does this mean?

Health care providers have the required knowledge and skills to work with adolescents, and to provide them with the required health services.

Why is this important?

Health care providers need to be competent in working with adolescents in general, in the 'adolescent-specific' aspects of providing health promotion, preventive, curative and rehabilitative services, as well as in interpersonal relations and communication.

18. Health care providers used evidence-based protocols and guidelines to provide health services

What does this mean?

Health service provision is based on protocols and guidelines that are technically sound and of proven usefulness. Ideally they should be adapted to the requirements of the national/sub-national situation and approved by the relevant authorities.

Why is this important?

In using such tools, health care providers are assured of the best course of action in responding to their adolescent patients.

19. Health care providers are able to devote adequate time to their patients

What does this mean?

Health care providers are able to dedicate sufficient time to deal effectively with their adolescent patients.

Why is this important?

This is important for two reasons: firstly, adolescents may find it difficult to communicate, be shy or frightened and may need extra time and encouragement to talk about their real concerns; and secondly, because health care providers need adequate time to deal with their patients in an effective manner.

20. Points of health service delivery have the necessary equipment, supplies and basic services to deliver the required health services

What does this mean?

Each point of health service delivery has the necessary equipment, supplies (including medicines) and basic services (e.g. water and sanitation) needed to deliver essential health services.

Why is this important?

Without the basic materials, health services cannot be provided effectively. The provision of health services in such a context may even endanger the health of adolescents.

ANNEX 2

A menu of complementary actions at national, district and local levels to ensure that characteristics of adolescent-friendly health services are achieved

Characteristics of adolescent-friendly health services	Actions to be taken at the national level	Actions to be taken at the district level	Actions to be taken at the health service delivery point (HSDP)
Actions to make HSDPs more equitable			
Policies and procedures are in place that do not restrict the provision of health services	– National officials to review laws and policies; and modify existing ones where they restrict the provision of health services. – National officials to communicate laws and policies to relevant officials at district level.	– District officials to communicate laws and policies to HSDP managers. – District officials to support the formulation of procedures for HSDP managers, in line with these laws and policies.	– Manager to work with service providers and support staff to ensure that the procedures are applied.
Health care providers treat all adolescent clients with equal care and respect, regardless of status	– National officials to communicate the importance of avoiding discrimination to district officials. – National officials to ensure that preventing discrimination is addressed in training materials and in handbooks..	– District officials to communicate to HSDP managers of the importance of preventing discrimination. – District officials to work with HSDP managers to identify groups of adolescents who could be discriminated against. – District officials to encourage HSDP managers to be alert to the occurrence of discrimination and to take corrective actions if and when it does happen.	– Manager to work with service providers and support staff to identify groups of adolescents who could be discriminated against. – Manager to communicate the importance of avoiding discrimination. – Manager to be alert to the occurrence of discrimination and to take corrective actions if and when it does happen.
Support staff treat all adolescent clients with equal care and respect, regardless of status	-"-	-"-	-"-
Actions to make HSDPs more accessible			
Policies and procedures are in place that ensure that health services are either free or affordable to adolescents	– National officials to review laws and policies; and modify existing ones to ensure that health services are free or affordable to adolescents. – National officials to communicate laws and policies to relevant officials at district level.	– District officials to communicate laws and policies to HSDP managers. – District officials to support the formulation of procedures for HSDP managers, in line with these laws and policies.	– Manager to work with service providers and support staff to ensure that the procedures are applied.
The HSDP has convenient working hours	– National officials to communicate the importance of local actions (i.e. modifying working hours to meet the needs of specific groups of adolescents) to address this issue.	– District officials to communicate the importance of local actions (i.e. modifying working hours to meet the needs of specific groups of adolescents) to address this issue, to HSDP managers.	– Manager to work with service providers and support staff to determine whether the working hours could be modified to take into account the needs of specific groups of adolescents.

Characteristics of adolescent-friendly health services	Actions to be taken at the national level	Actions to be taken at the district level	Actions to be taken at the health service delivery point (HSDP)
Adolescents are well informed about the range of reproductive health services available and how to obtain them	– National officials to communicate the need for district officials and HSDP managers to take actions to help inform adolescents about the range of health services that are be provided at HSDP.	– District officials to communicate what health services are provided, where and when they are provided, and how much they cost: (i) in the mass media (where possible); (ii) in meetings with representatives of other sectors (e.g. education) and civil society institutions (e.g. NGOs); – District officials to communicate the importance of local action (i.e. putting up a notice board) to address this issue, to HSDP managers.	– Manager to carry out the following actions: (i) Put up a notice board indicating what health services are provided, when they are provided, and how much they cost; (ii) Prepare a leaflet indicating what health services are provided, when they are provided, and how much they cost.
Community members understand the benefits that adolescents will gain by obtaining the health services they need, and support their provision	– National officials to communicate the rationale for providing health services to adolescents in the mass media, and in meetings with national-level representatives of other sectors (e.g. education) and civil society institutions (e.g. religious bodies) – National officials to communicate the need for district officials to communicate this message to – district-level representatives of other sectors (e.g. education) and civil society institutions (e.g. NGOs).	– District officials to communicate the rationale for providing health services to adolescents in meetings with district-level representatives of other sectors (e.g. education) and civil society institutions (e.g. NGOs).	– Manager and staff (including service providers and support staff) to identify key institutions in the catchment area of the HSDP, and to meet with heads of these institutions to explain them, the rationale for providing health services to adolescents.

Characteristics of adolescent-friendly health services	Actions to be taken at the national level	Actions to be taken at the district level	Actions to be taken at the health service delivery point (HSDP)
Some health services and health-related commodities are provided to adolescents in the community by selected community members, outreach workers and adolescents themselves	– National officials to communicate the importance of reaching out to selected groups of adolescents in the community with selected health services (e.g. some aspects of antenatal care) and commodities (e.g. iron and folic acid tablets).	– District officials to communicate the importance of outreach activities and/or working with NGOs in the community that could engage selected adults or adolescents to provide health services and commodities to adolescents in the community. – District officials to work with HSDP managers to identify which groups of adolescents to reach, where to reach them, and what health services and commodities to reach them with.	– Manager to set aside some time from selected staff members for outreach work. – Manager and staff to identify NGOs which could engage selected adults and adolescents to provide health services and commodities to adolescents in the community.
Actions to make HSDPs more acceptable			
Policies and procedures are in place that guarantee client confidentiality	– National officials to: (i) clearly outline the events/conditions service providers are required to report to the relevant authorities (such as sexual assault, road traffic accidents and gunshot wounds); (ii) communicate that in all other circumstances, HSDP managers, service providers and support staff are required to maintain the confidentiality of their adolescent clients. – National officials to outline clear procedures to be followed in HSDP to ensure that information about clients is not disclosed to third parties, and that client records are held securely.	– District officials to ensure that HSDP managers are aware of the national policy on confidentiality and the procedures to translate these policies into action. – District officials to communicate the importance of applying these procedures.	– Managers to work with service providers and support staff to ensure that they are all aware of the policies and recommended procedures. – Managers to ensure that the recommended procedures are translated into concrete actions with clear designation of responsibilities within the HSDP.
Point of service delivery ensures privacy	– National officials to communicate the importance of actions to ensure visual and auditory privacy during registration and during consultation with a service provider.	– District officials to communicate the importance of ensuring visual and auditory privacy, and to support managers in making any modifications that are needed to HSDPs to ensure this.	– Managers to work with service providers and support staff to determine what could be done to ensure both visual and auditory privacy in the HSDP, given the prevailing resource constraints.

Characteristics of adolescent-friendly health services	Actions to be taken at the national level	Actions to be taken at the district level	Actions to be taken at the health service delivery point (HSDP)
Health care providers are non-judgmental, considerate, and easy to relate to	– National officials to communicate the importance of these attributes among health care providers and support staff. – National officials to ensure that these issues are addressed in training materials and in handbooks.	– District officials to conduct workshops to orient/train HSDP managers, health care providers and support staff. – District officials to encourage HSDP managers to support health care providers and support staff in being non-judgemental and considerate, and to relate to their adolescents in a friendly manner; and where appropriate to take corrective actions when needed.	– Managers to communicate to health care providers and support staff about the importance of being non-judgemental and considerate, and to relate to adolescent clients in a friendly manner. – Managers to be alert to breaches of this, and to take corrective actions.
Point of service delivery ensures consultations occur in a short waiting time, with or without an appointment, and (where necessary) swift referral	– National officials to communicate the importance of actions to keep waiting times as short as possible and to ensure that referral mechanisms are in place and function well.	– District officials to work with HSDP managers in the district, to set up/strengthen referral mechanisms.	– Managers to work with service providers and support staff to determine what could be done to keep waiting times as short as possible. – Managers to ensure that service providers and support staff are aware of, and apply, referral mechanisms to providers of health and social services.
Point of service delivery has an appealing and clean environment	– National officials to communicate the importance of actions to make the physical environment of HSDPs appealing and clean.	– District officials to encourage HSDP managers to take the needed actions to make the physical environment appealing and clean.	– Managers to work with service providers and support staff to make the physical environment of the HSDP (e.g. to have adequate and comfortable seats in the waiting area) and clean (e.g. to ensure that the toilets are clean and that drinking water and is available).
Point of service delivery provides information and education through a variety of channels	– National officials to develop informational/educational materials and send them to the districts. – National officials to liaise with NGOs working on adolescent health issues in the country to explore whether the materials they produce could be displayed/disseminated to the districts.	– District officials to arrange for the delivery of informational/educational materials obtained from national officials or NGOs, to HSDPs. – District officials to liaise with NGOs working in their district to explore whether the materials they produce could be displayed and disseminated by HDSPs.	– Managers to ensure that educational/informational materials are displayed/distributed. – Even if no materials are obtained from district officials, managers to work with service providers to ensure that clipping from newspapers and magazines, and hand-made materials are displayed.

Characteristics of adolescent-friendly health services	Actions to be taken at the national level	Actions to be taken at the district level	Actions to be taken at the health service delivery point (HSDP)
Adolescents are actively involved in designing, assessing and providing health services	– National officials to communicate the importance of involving adolescents in designing, assessing and providing health services.	– District officials to encourage HSDP managers to involve adolescents in designing, assessing and providing health services.	– Managers to work with service providers and support staff to identify and draw in adolescents employed by organizations working with young people or volunteers from the community into the work of the HSDP: (i) by drawing upon their ideas and suggestions in designing health service provision; (ii) by involving them in assessing and providing health services.
Actions to ensure that the health services provided are appropriate			
The required package of health care is provided to fulfil the needs of all adolescents either at the point of service delivery or through referral linkages	– National officials to list the health services that are to be provided at each level (e.g. primary level, secondary level and referral level).	– District officials to work with HSDP managers ensure that HSDPs provide all the health services that they are required to, and to facilitate access to those that they do not provide with referral linkages.	– Managers to ensure that HSDPs provide all the health services they are required to, and facilitate access to those they do not provide with referral linkages to other HSDPs.
Actions to ensure that health services provided effectively			
Health care providers have the required competencies to work with adolescents and to provide them with the required health services	– National officials need to develop teaching/learning materials to build the competencies of service providers to deliver the required based on a needs assessment. – National officials to develop/adapt a handy desk reference tool for service providers. – National officials to set up a system for supportive supervision. (It would be useful if that includes elements of self assessment, peer assessment, supervisor assessment and external assessment).	– District officials to work with HSDP managers to ensure that service providers in the district undergo training/orientation. – District officials to supply HSDP managers with desk reference tools to service providers. – District officials support HSDP managers to put in place self, peer and supervisor assessment systems; and to put in place an external assessment system.	– Managers to ensure that: (i) service providers are trained/oriented; (ii) services providers have desk reference tools; (iii) self, peer and supervisor assessments are carried out in the context of supportive supervision.
Health care providers use evidence-based protocols and guidelines to provide health services	– National authorities to develop evidence-based protocols and guidelines. – National authorities to ensure that these protocols and guidelines are included in teaching/learning materials and desk reference tools.	-"-	-"-

Making health services adolescent friendly

Characteristics of adolescent-friendly health services	Actions to be taken at the national level	Actions to be taken at the district level	Actions to be taken at the health service delivery point (HSDP)
Health care providers are able to dedicate sufficient time to deal effectively with their adolescent clients	– National authorities to communicate the importance of this characteristic.	– District officials to communicate the importance of this characteristic to HSDP managers. – District officials to support HSDP managers to 'spread out' the clinics provided at the HSDP (e.g. antenatal clinic) and deploy staff in a way that reduces crowding in the waiting area and pressure on service providers to 'dispose of' patients quickly.	– Managers to work with service providers and support staff to identify how best to spread out the clinics provided at the HSDP and to deploy staff in way that contribute in spreading the patient load through the working hours of the HSDP. – Managers to encourage service providers to devote adequate time to each patient.
The HSDP has the required equipment, supplies, and basic services necessary to deliver the required health services	– National officials to prepare lists of equipment and supplies that HSDPs need to have to provide the stipulated package of health services. – National officials to send these lists to district officials. – National officials to work with district officials to determine what equipment and what stocks of supplies are required to provide the stipulated package of health services; and to ensure that they are sent out on in good time.	– District officials to give HSDP managers the list of equipment and supplies that HSDPs need to have to provide the stipulated package of health services. – District officials to work with HSDP managers to determine what equipment and what quantities of supplies are required on a monthly/quarterly basis. – District officials to work with national officials to obtain the equipment and supplies required by the district in good time.	– Managers to have at-hand lists of equipment and supplies that are needed to provide the stipulated package of health services. – Managers to work with service providers and support staff to put in place a system to review if the pieces of equipment are in good order and that the stocks of supplies are adequate. – Managers to organize regular servicing/repairs of equipment and to ensure that adequate stocks of supplies are maintained.